Embrace Your Essence: 101 Self-Care Practices for Busy Moms

Copyright © 2024 by Carole Valluy

Table of Contents

Introduction: Awakening to Self-Care

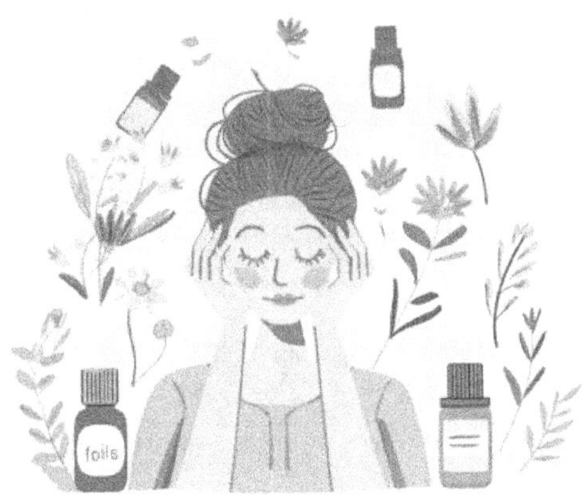

In the stillness of an early morning, when the world whispers the promise of a new day, a profound realization awaits—self-care is not just an act of personal kindness; it's a necessity for every mom navigating the beautiful, yet often overwhelming, journey of motherhood. I am Carole Valluy, and I've walked the path you're on, balancing the demands of family, work, and personal aspirations, all the while forgetting the one person who needed care the most—myself.

This book, **"Embrace Your Essence: 101 Self-Care Practices for Busy Moms,"** is born from my journey and the shared experiences of countless moms I've had the privilege to connect with. It's a guide, a companion, and a gentle reminder that amidst the chaos of schedules, deadlines, and commitments, your well-being is paramount.

Why self-care, you might ask? The answer lies in the very essence of our daily lives. As moms, we are accustomed to putting others first, often at the expense of our health and happiness. We wear our exhaustion like badges of honor, believing that the more we sacrifice, the better moms we become. But this couldn't be further from the truth. Neglecting our well-being doesn't make us better parents; it leaves us drained, stressed, and disconnected from the joy of motherhood.

Self-care is the antidote to this cycle of exhaustion. It's about reclaiming your vitality, peace, and joy. It's about recognizing that you, too, deserve the love and attention you so freely give to others. This book is not about grand gestures of self-indulgence but about simple, practical practices that weave into the fabric of your everyday life, making self-care accessible and achievable for every mom, no matter how busy.

As we begin this journey together, I invite you to open your heart to the possibility of transformation. The practices within these pages are designed to guide you gently toward a more balanced, fulfilled, and joyful life. From quick wins for busy days to nurturing your body, mind, and soul, we will explore the multifaceted aspects of self-care, tailored specifically for the unique challenges and blessings of motherhood.

This is not a journey you have to undertake alone. Throughout this book, I share not only practical advice but also personal anecdotes and stories from other moms, creating a tapestry of shared experiences and collective wisdom. Together, we will navigate the path of self-care, learning to prioritize our well-being with the same passion and dedication we give to our families.

As you turn these pages, remember that self-care is a personal and evolving journey. What works for one may not work for another, and that's okay. This book is designed to be a resource you can return to time and again, finding new practices that resonate with your changing needs and circumstances.

So, dear reader, as the dawn breaks and you step into the day ahead, remember that the journey to embracing your essence begins with a simple act of self-care. Let this book be your guide, your inspiration, and a reminder that in the world of motherhood, you are not alone. Together, let's awaken to self-care and rediscover the joy, peace, and fulfillment that come from nurturing ourselves.

Welcome to "Embrace Your Essence: 101 Self-Care Practices for Busy Moms." Welcome to the beginning of a beautiful journey toward embracing your true essence.

Author

Carole Valluy

Chapter 1: The Foundation of Self-Care

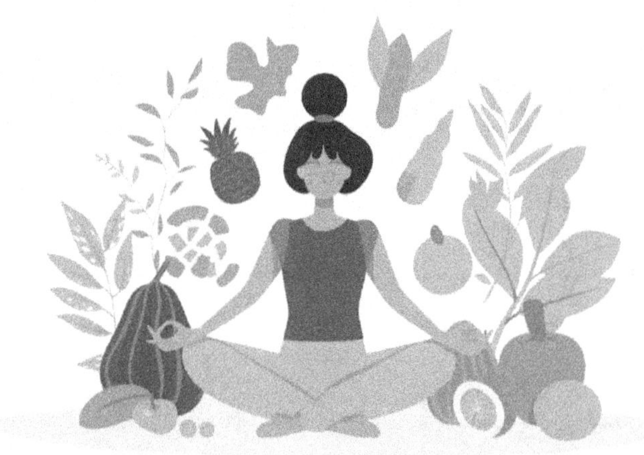

As the first light of dawn creeps through the curtains, casting a warm glow across the room, it serves as a gentle reminder of the world's natural rhythm and the importance of aligning our self-care practices with our personal needs. In the quiet moments before the day begins, we find a precious opportunity to reflect on what self-care truly means and how it forms the foundation of our well-being. This chapter is dedicated to helping you, the busy mom, understand and embrace self-care not as a luxury, but as a necessity.

Understanding Self-Care: Beyond the Basics

Self-care is often portrayed as a series of indulgent activities—a bubble bath, a spa day, or an extravagant shopping spree. While these can be part of self-care, at its core, self-care is about much more. It's about nurturing yourself in a way that keeps you grounded, balanced, and feeling fulfilled. It involves attending to your physical, emotional, mental, and spiritual needs in a manner that fuels you to be your best self for you and those you love.

Identifying Your Needs: Physical, Emotional, Mental, and Spiritual

1. Physical Needs: Your physical body is the vessel that carries you through life. It's essential to listen to its needs, which include nutrition, hydration, rest, and movement. A simple practice to start with is tuning in to your body's signals. Are you thirsty? Are you tired? Learning to respond to these signals promptly can significantly enhance your physical well-being.

2. Emotional Needs: Emotional self-care involves processing your feelings, seeking positive relationships, and finding healthy outlets for stress and anger. One initial step could be implementing a daily check-in with yourself. How are you feeling today? Acknowledging your emotions is the first step toward managing them effectively.

3. Mental Needs: Your mental health is just as crucial as your physical health. Mental self-care can include anything that keeps your mind sharp and your stress levels in check. This might involve setting aside time for activities that challenge your brain or simply ensuring you have moments of quiet to prevent mental overload.

4. Spiritual Needs: Regardless of religious belief, spiritual self-care is about connecting with what gives your life meaning and purpose. It can be as simple as spending time in nature, meditating, or practicing gratitude. Finding what uplifts your spirit is a deeply personal journey and a fundamental aspect of self-care.

Creating Your Personal Self-Care Plan

A personal self-care plan is a tailored approach to addressing your unique needs. It's not about creating a rigid schedule that adds more stress to your life but about integrating self-care into your daily routine in a way that feels natural and fulfilling. Here's how to start:

Step 1: Assessment Take a moment to assess your current self-care practices. What are you already doing that serves your well-being? What areas are you neglecting? This honest appraisal is your starting point.

Step 2: Prioritization Not all self-care practices are created equal. Some will be more relevant and beneficial to you than others. Prioritize the practices that address your most pressing needs first.

Step 3: Integration Look at your typical day and see where you can integrate self-care practices without overwhelming yourself. Can you listen to an audiobook during your commute for mental stimulation? Or perhaps you can practice deep breathing exercises before starting your day for emotional balance.

Step 4: Flexibility Your self-care plan should be flexible. Some days you might have only five minutes to spare, and that's okay. Self-care is about doing what you can, when you can.

Step 5: Review and Adjust Regularly review your self-care plan. What's working? What isn't? Your needs will change over time, and so should your self-care practices.

Quick Wins for Busy Days

We all have those days when 24 hours simply don't seem enough. Here are some quick self-care practices that can fit into even the busiest schedules:

1. Five-Minute Mindfulness Techniques:

- **Breathing Space:** Take a five-minute break to focus solely on your breath. Breathe in for four counts, hold for four counts, and exhale for four counts. This simple practice can center your thoughts and reduce stress.

2. The Art of Deep Breathing Exercises:

- **4-7-8 Technique:** Breathe in for 4 seconds, hold your breath for 7 seconds, and exhale slowly for 8 seconds. This technique is especially beneficial before sleep.

3. Energizing Stretch Routines for Every Mom:

- **Morning Stretch:** Before getting out of bed, spend a few minutes stretching your body to awaken your muscles and boost your energy for the day ahead.

These practices are not time-consuming but can have a profound impact on your well-being. The key is consistency. Even on your busiest days, dedicating a few minutes to self-care can make a significant difference in how you feel and how you navigate the challenges of motherhood.

Exploring Self-Care as a Journey

Embarking on a self-care journey is a courageous step toward recognizing your worth and acknowledging that you deserve to be cared for, just as you care for others. This chapter has laid the groundwork for understanding and integrating self-care into your life. Remember, self-care is not selfish; it's essential. By taking care of yourself, you're not only enhancing your own well-being but also enriching the lives of those around you with your best self.

Chapter 2: Quick Wins for Busy Days

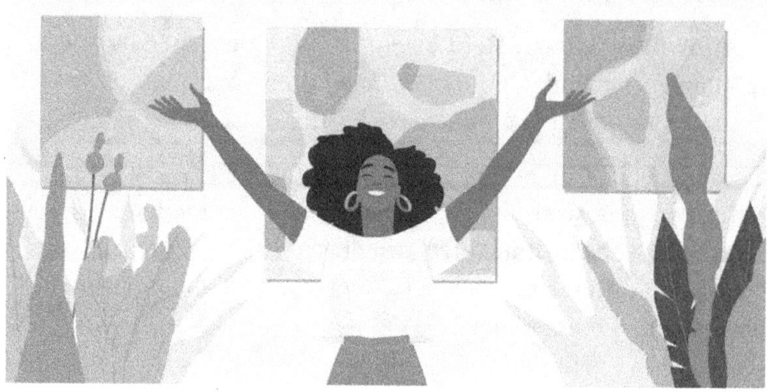

In the symphony of life, busy moms are the conductors, orchestrating a delicate balance of needs, wants, and must-dos. Yet, amid the cacophony of daily obligations, finding moments for self-care can seem an insurmountable task. It's in these bustling times that the magic of quick, effective self-care practices shines brightest, offering a beacon of rejuvenation for those who feel they barely have a moment to breathe. This chapter delves into the art of carving out pockets of peace and vitality, ensuring that even on your busiest days, self-care remains a non-negotiable part of your routine.

Five-Minute Mindfulness Techniques

1. **One-Minute Breathing:** Begin by finding a comfortable seated position, close your eyes, and focus solely on your breath for one full minute. Inhale deeply through your nose, allowing your chest and belly to rise, and exhale slowly through your mouth. This practice can serve as a grounding technique, bringing you back to the present moment and reducing stress.

2. **Sensory Grounding:** Engage each of your senses sequentially. Look for five things you can see, four you can touch, three you can hear, two you can smell, and one you can taste. This quick sensory check-in can help distract from anxiety and center your thoughts.

3. **Gratitude Reflection:** Take a minute to silently acknowledge three things you're grateful for. Gratitude can shift your mindset from scarcity to abundance, making challenges seem more manageable.

4. **Mindful Sipping:** Whether it's a morning coffee or a glass of water, focus entirely on the act of sipping your drink. Notice the temperature, the taste, and the sensation as you drink. This practice can transform a mundane activity into a moment of mindfulness.

5. **Visualized Breathing:** Close your eyes and imagine a serene setting. With each inhale, visualize peace flowing into your body, and with each exhale, imagine stress leaving. This visualization helps create a mental escape, offering a brief respite from the day's demands.

The Art of Deep Breathing Exercises

6. **Diaphragmatic Breathing:** Lie down or sit comfortably, place one hand on your belly, and breathe deeply into your diaphragm (not just your chest), feeling your hand rise and fall. This encourages full oxygen exchange and can decrease the stress hormone cortisol.

7. **4-7-8 Breathing:** Inhale quietly through your nose for 4 seconds, hold your breath for 7 seconds, and exhale forcefully through your mouth for 8 seconds. This exercise promotes relaxation and can aid in falling asleep more quickly.

8. **Box Breathing:** Inhale for 4 seconds, hold for 4 seconds, exhale for 4 seconds, and hold again for 4 seconds. This method is used by athletes and military personnel to calm nerves and focus the mind.

9. **Alternate Nostril Breathing:** Close off one nostril with a finger, inhale through the open nostril, close it off, then exhale through the other nostril. This practice is said to harmonize the two hemispheres of the brain, resulting in emotional balance and mental clarity.

10. **Progressive Muscle Relaxation:** Tense each muscle group in your body for about five seconds and then relax for 30 seconds, working your way from your toes to your head. This technique reduces physical tension and mental stress simultaneously.

Energizing Stretch Routines for Every Mom

11. **Neck and Shoulder Release:** Tilt your head from side to side, bringing your ear close to your shoulder, and gently roll your shoulders backward and forward. This releases tension accumulated from daily activities like driving or sitting at a desk.

12. **Spinal Twist:** Sitting on a chair, place your right hand on your left knee and gently twist your torso to the left, looking over your left shoulder. Repeat on the opposite side. This stretch can invigorate your spine and refresh your energy levels.

13. **Forward Fold:** Stand with feet hip-width apart, exhale, and fold forward from your hips, reaching towards the ground. This pose helps relieve stress, stretches your hamstrings, and revitalizes your circulation.

14. **Cat-Cow Stretch:** On all fours, inhale as you arch your back, looking up (cow), and exhale as you round your spine, tucking your chin to your chest (cat). This movement increases spinal flexibility and can ease tension in your back.

15. **Legs-Up-the-Wall:** Lie on your back and extend your legs up against a wall. This passive inversion helps drain lymph and refreshes the legs and feet, offering a quick rejuvenation for those who spend a lot of time standing or walking.

These fifteen practices are designed to be seamlessly integrated into the busiest of days, ensuring that self-care is not only attainable but also effective. They serve as a testament to the idea that self-care does not need to be time-consuming or elaborate; sometimes, the simplest acts can have the most profound impact on our well-being.

Engaging in these quick self-care practices can significantly improve your mood, energy levels, and overall sense of balance, proving that even the busiest moms can carve out moments of serenity in their day. By adopting these practices, you affirm the importance of your well-being, recognizing that taking care of yourself is not just a luxury—it's a necessity for continuing to care for others with love and energy.

Remember, the goal of integrating these practices into your life is not to add more to your already full plate but to offer you small oases of calm and rejuvenation amidst the chaos. Whether it's through a minute of deep breathing, a quick stretch, or a moment of mindful sipping, each practice is a step towards embracing self-care as a vital component of your daily routine. In doing so, you not only enhance your own life but also set a powerful example for those around you, illustrating the transformative power of taking small moments for oneself, even on the busiest of days.

Chapter 3: Nourishing Your Body

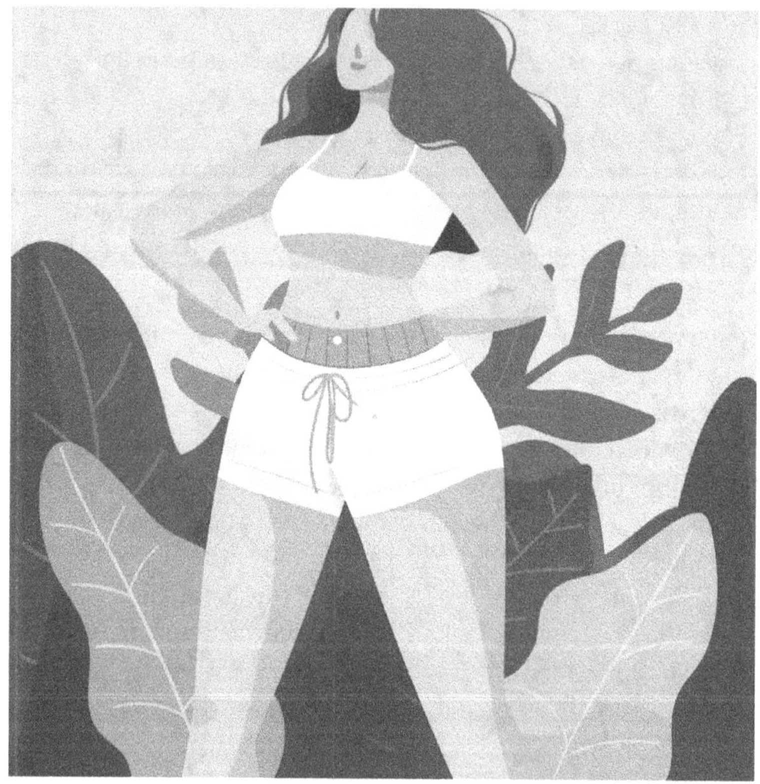

In the tapestry of self-care, nourishing your body is akin to selecting the finest threads to weave your well-being. It's about more than just eating right; it's a holistic approach to fueling your life force, ensuring every cell in your body vibrates with energy and health. For busy moms, the challenge isn't just about making healthy choices; it's about integrating these choices seamlessly into a life that often feels like it's running on fast-forward. This chapter is dedicated to transforming the necessity of nourishment into an art form that fits into the crevices of your packed schedule.

Simplifying Healthy Eating for Busy Schedules

1. Planning is Your Power Tool: The cornerstone of simplifying healthy eating lies in planning. Dedicate a time each week to plan your meals. This doesn't have to be a laborious process; even jotting down a rough guide on your phone while waiting for your kids at soccer practice can work wonders.

2. Batch Cooking and Prep: Consider preparing components of your meals in advance. Cooking a large batch of quinoa on Sunday, for example, can provide a versatile base for meals throughout the week. Similarly, chopping vegetables in advance can save precious minutes during the weekday hustle.

3. Healthy Eating Kits: Create your own "healthy eating kits" for emergencies. These can include pre-portioned nuts, seeds, and dried fruits, along with whole grain crackers and nut butter. Having these at hand can prevent the all-too-common vending machine dash.

4. Embrace Freezing: Your freezer is an underrated hero in the quest for healthy eating. Freezing portions of cooked meals not only preserves their nutritional value but also means you always have something healthy on standby.

5. Smart Snacking: Choose snacks that are both satisfying and nutritious. A piece of fruit with a handful of nuts, Greek yogurt with a sprinkle of granola, or a smoothie can provide the energy boost you need without the sugar crash.

Hydration: The Essence of Vitality

6. Start Your Day with Water: Begin each morning by drinking a glass of water. Overnight, your body becomes naturally dehydrated; replenishing your fluids kick-starts your metabolism and brain function.

7. Infuse Flavor: If you find plain water unappealing, infuse it with fruits, cucumbers, or herbs. A pitcher of water with lemon and mint or berries can be both refreshing and enticing.

8. Hydration Reminders: In the digital age, let technology assist you. Apps that remind you to drink water or even setting simple alarms can help maintain your hydration levels throughout the day.

9. Eat Your Water: Remember, hydration doesn't just come from what you drink. Consuming fruits and vegetables with high water content, like cucumbers, tomatoes, oranges, and watermelons, can also contribute to your daily fluid intake.

10. The Right Mug: Invest in a water bottle or mug that you love. It's a simple trick, but having a vessel that is both convenient and pleasing to the eye can encourage you to drink more water.

Sleep Rituals for Restorative Nights

11. Wind-Down Routine: Establish a wind-down routine before bed to signal to your body that it's time to rest. This could be as simple as a cup of herbal tea, reading a book, or practicing a few minutes of gentle yoga.

12. Digital Detox: Aim to turn off all digital devices at least an hour before bedtime. The blue light emitted by screens can disrupt your circadian rhythm and interfere with the production of melatonin, the hormone responsible for sleep.

13. Comfort is Key: Invest in making your sleeping environment as comfortable as possible. This means finding the right mattress and pillows, and ensuring your room is cool, dark, and quiet.

14. Aromatherapy: Utilize the power of aromatherapy to enhance your sleep quality. Lavender oil is renowned for its relaxing properties; a few drops on your pillow or in a diffuser can work wonders.

15. Mindful Breathing: Engage in mindful breathing or meditation to calm your mind before sleep. Techniques such as the 4-7-8 method, where you breathe in for 4 seconds, hold for 7 seconds, and exhale for 8 seconds, can be particularly effective.

By integrating these practices into your daily routine, you not only nourish your body but also enrich your soul, weaving a tapestry of health that extends beyond the dinner plate. Remember, the essence of self-care is in the simplicity and sustainability of your choices. Choose practices that resonate with you and fit into your life seamlessly, allowing you to embrace the journey of nourishment with joy and ease.

Chapter 4: Cultivating Emotional Resilience

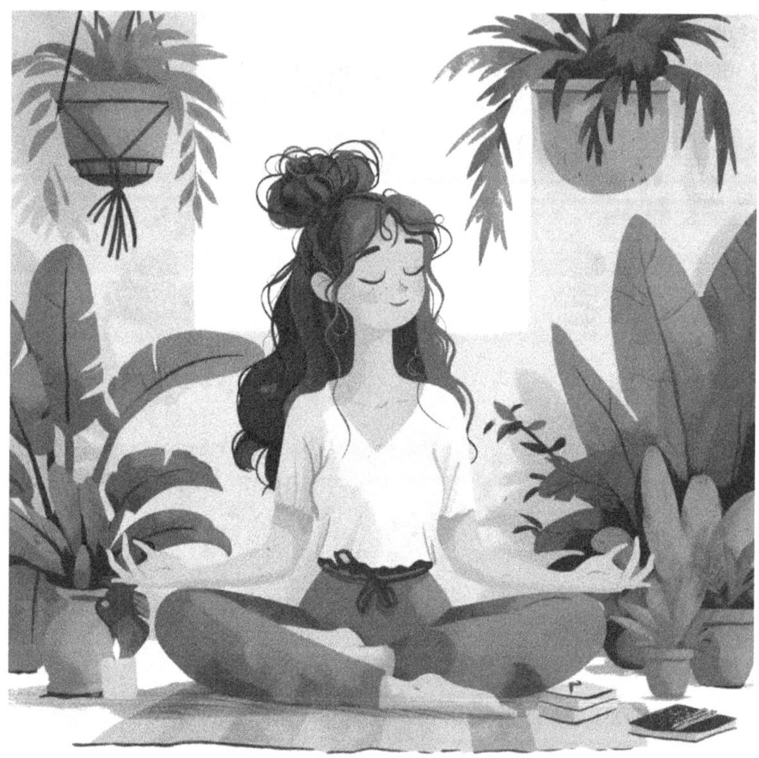

In the quiet moments before dawn, when the world is still asleep and the first light of day has yet to break, lies a sacred opportunity for reflection and emotional grounding. For busy moms, these moments are precious and few, yet they hold the key to cultivating a resilience that can weather any storm. Emotional resilience is not about avoiding feelings or pretending that challenges don't exist; it's about facing them head-on with grace, understanding, and an unwavering strength that comes from within.

Emotional Journaling for Clarity and Strength

Emotional journaling is a powerful tool for cultivating emotional resilience. It provides a private, non-judgmental space to express feelings, reflect on experiences, and clarify thoughts. Start with just five minutes a day, writing freely about anything that comes to mind. Focus on how you felt during the day's events, what triggered these feelings, and how you responded. Over time, you'll begin to notice patterns and triggers, giving you insight into how to manage your emotions more effectively.

1. **Gratitude Journaling:** Begin or end each day by writing down three things you're grateful for. This practice shifts focus from what's lacking to what's abundant in your life, fostering positivity and resilience.

2. **Emotion Tracking:** Dedicate a section of your journal to track your emotions throughout the day. Use colors, symbols, or words to describe how you felt at different times. This visual representation can help you identify what brings you joy and what drains your energy.

3. **Letter Writing:** Write letters you never intend to send. Address them to people who have hurt you, to loved ones who have passed, or even to yourself. This exercise can be incredibly cathartic, helping to release pent-up emotions and find closure.

4. **Future Scripting:** Write about your future, focusing on your hopes and dreams. Describe in detail how you feel having achieved these dreams. This practice can help align your present actions with your future goals, providing motivation and a sense of purpose.

5. **Problem-Solving Entries:** When faced with a challenge, use your journal to brainstorm potential solutions. Writing down your problems and possible solutions can make them seem more manageable and less daunting.

Building a Supportive Community

A **supportive community** plays a crucial role in emotional resilience. Surrounding yourself with people who uplift and understand you can provide a buffer against life's challenges.

1. **Join or Create a Support Group:** Whether it's a formal group for moms or an informal gathering of friends, sharing experiences and advice can be incredibly supportive. Platforms like Meetup or Facebook can help you find local groups or even online communities that resonate with your needs.

2. **Family Meetings:** Regular family meetings can strengthen bonds and improve communication. Use this time to express needs, share feelings, and discuss how to support each other. It's a practice that models emotional resilience for your children, showing them the importance of openness and support.

3. **Partner Check-Ins:** Schedule weekly check-ins with your partner to discuss your emotional well-being. This dedicated time encourages mutual support and understanding, reinforcing your partnership as a source of strength.

4. **Mentorship:** Seek out a mentor who embodies resilience and emotional wisdom. This could be someone from your professional network, a personal acquaintance, or even a counselor or therapist. Their guidance can offer valuable perspectives and coping strategies.

5. **Volunteer Work:** Engaging in volunteer work can expand your support network and connect you with like-minded individuals. It also provides a sense of purpose and fulfillment, which are key components of emotional resilience.

Techniques for Managing Stress and Anxiety

Stress and anxiety are common challenges for busy moms, but with the right techniques, they can be managed effectively, fostering emotional resilience.

1. **Deep Breathing Exercises:** Simple yet powerful, deep breathing can calm the mind and reduce stress. Practice the 4-7-8 technique: inhale for 4 seconds, hold for 7 seconds, and exhale for 8 seconds. This exercise can quickly help bring your focus back to the present moment, reducing anxiety.

2. **Progressive Muscle Relaxation (PMR):** PMR involves tensing each muscle group in the body tightly, but not to the point of strain, and then slowly relaxing them. This practice can help you become more aware of physical sensations and reduce stress levels.

3. **Mindfulness Meditation:** Dedicate a few minutes each day to mindfulness meditation. Sit quietly, focus on your breath, and observe your thoughts and feelings without judgment. This practice can help you develop a calm and non-reactive mindset.

4. **Visualization:** Take a moment to visualize a place that brings you peace. It could be a beach, a forest, or any setting that calms you. Engage all your senses in this visualization to enhance its calming effect.

5. **Setting Realistic Goals:** Often, stress arises from feeling overwhelmed by unrealistic expectations. Break down your tasks into manageable steps and set achievable goals. Celebrate small victories to motivate yourself and reduce anxiety.

Cultivating emotional resilience is a journey that requires patience, practice, and persistence. Through emotional journaling, building a supportive community, and employing techniques to manage stress and anxiety, busy moms can forge a path to a more balanced and resilient life. It's about embracing the full spectrum of your emotions, learning from them, and finding strength in vulnerability. Remember, resilience is not a destination but a way of traveling through life's ups and downs with grace, courage, and an unwavering belief in yourself.

Chapter 5: Fostering Mental Well-Being

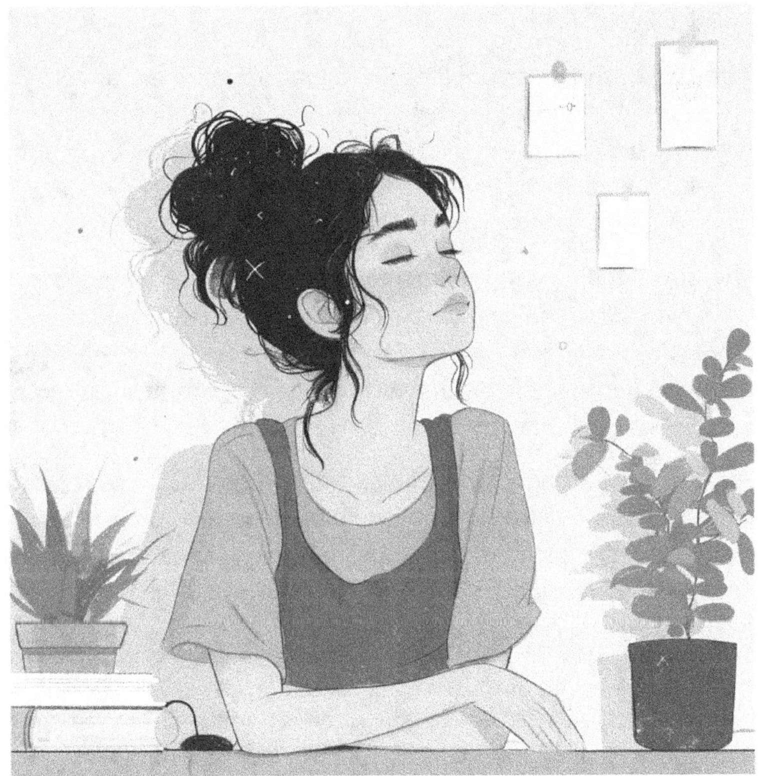

As dawn breaks, casting a gentle glow through your window, the world outside begins to stir, and so does your mind. It's a canvas, fresh and ready for the day's brush strokes. Yet, for many, this canvas can quickly become cluttered with the demands of motherhood, work, and daily life, leaving little room for peace and creativity. This chapter is your guide to reclaiming that canvas, transforming it into a masterpiece of mental well-being through mindfulness, digital detox, and continuous engagement of the mind.

Mindfulness: Embracing the Present

The Practice of Mindful Mornings: Start your day by grounding yourself in the now. Before the rush begins, spend five minutes in silence, observing the morning light, the coolness of the air, or the quiet hum of the world around you. This practice helps set a calm tone for the day ahead.

Mindful Eating: Turn meals into an exercise of mindfulness by focusing fully on the experience of eating. Notice the colors, textures, and flavors of your food, appreciating each bite. This not only enhances the enjoyment of your meal but also promotes better digestion and satisfaction.

Walking Meditation: Incorporate mindfulness into your daily walk, whether it's taking the kids to school or a stroll around the block. Pay attention to each step, the rhythm of your breath, and the sights and sounds around you. This can transform a routine walk into a refreshing mental reset.

Mindful Listening: Practice being fully present in conversations, whether with your children, partner, or friends. Listen with the intent to understand, not to respond. This fosters deeper connections and helps you appreciate the nuances of your relationships.

Breathing Exercises for Stress: Whenever you feel overwhelmed, turn to focused breathing exercises. The 4-7-8 technique (inhale for 4 seconds, hold for 7, exhale for 8) is particularly effective in calming the mind and reducing stress levels.

Unplugging: The Art of Digital Detox

Set Screen-Free Times: Establish designated times of the day or week when you disconnect from all digital devices. This could be during meals, an hour before bedtime, or a screen-free Sunday. Use this time to connect with your family, dive into a book, or simply enjoy the tranquility of your surroundings.

Notification Management: Limit distractions by managing your notifications. Turn off non-essential alerts and designate specific times to check emails or social media. This reduces the constant pull to your devices, allowing you to focus more on the moment.

Digital Detox Challenges: Challenge yourself and your family to regular digital detoxes. Start with a few hours and gradually increase to a full day or weekend. Notice the difference in your stress levels, the quality of your interactions, and your overall sense of well-being.

Mindful Technology Use: When using technology, do so mindfully. Be intentional about your usage, choosing activities that add value to your life, such as educational apps, meditation guides, or fitness trackers. Avoid mindless scrolling, which can lead to increased anxiety and lost time.

Create Tech-Free Zones: Designate certain areas of your home, such as the bedroom or dining table, as tech-free zones. This encourages more face-to-face interactions with your family and ensures that technology does not dominate every aspect of your home life.

Lifelong Learning: Keeping the Mind Engaged

Pursue a Hobby: Engage your mind by picking up a new hobby or revisiting an old one. Whether it's painting, gardening, coding, or playing an instrument, hobbies provide a creative outlet and mental stimulation.

Read Regularly: Make reading a daily habit. Whether it's fiction, non-fiction, or professional development, reading expands your knowledge, vocabulary, and understanding of the world. It also offers an escape into different perspectives and stories.

Online Courses and Workshops: Take advantage of online learning platforms to explore new subjects or skills. Many offer free or low-cost courses that fit into a busy mom's schedule. This not only enhances your skill set but also keeps your mind active and engaged.

Join a Club or Group: Connect with others who share your interests by joining a book club, writing group, or local workshop. This provides social interaction, accountability, and the opportunity to learn from others.

Mindful Writing: Start a journal or blog to document your thoughts, experiences, and learnings. Writing is a powerful tool for self-expression and reflection, helping you process your emotions and ideas more clearly.

Cultivating a Mindful Environment at Home

Create Spaces for Relaxation: Designate a quiet corner in your home where you can retreat for meditation, reading, or simply to breathe. Equip this space with comforting items like cushions, a soft blanket, or calming scents.

Foster Open Communication: Encourage open and mindful communication within your family. Establish regular family meetings or check-ins where everyone can share their thoughts, feelings, and experiences without judgment.

Practice Gratitude: Implement a daily gratitude practice with your family. Share three things you're grateful for at the dinner table or keep a family gratitude journal. This shifts focus to the positive, enhancing everyone's mental well-being.

Model Mindfulness for Your Children: Children learn by example. By practicing mindfulness yourself, you teach your children the importance of living in the present, managing stress, and appreciating the simple joys of life.

Fostering mental well-being is a journey that starts with small steps. By integrating mindfulness practices, taking breaks from digital devices, and continuously engaging your mind in new learnings, you can navigate the complexities of motherhood with a sense of calm and resilience. Remember, the state of your mental health not only impacts you but also the atmosphere of your home and the well-being of your family. Embrace these practices as part of your daily life, and watch as your mental canvas becomes a vibrant tapestry of well-being, creativity, and joy.

Chapter 6: Spiritual Self-Care for Inner Peace

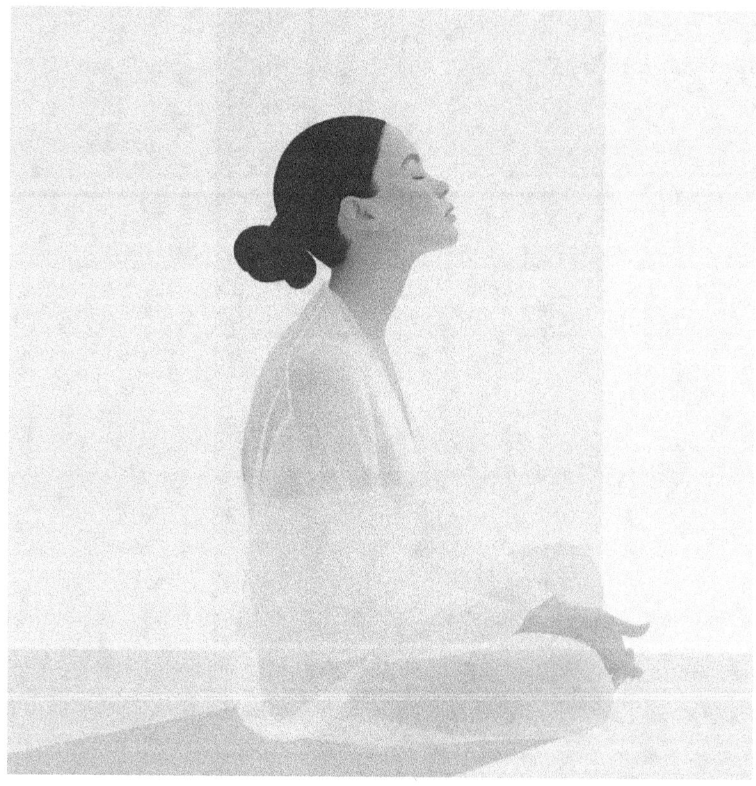

"In the stillness of the morning, before the world awakens, lies a sacred space for renewal and connection."

As a busy mom, finding moments of tranquility can seem like a distant dream. Yet, it is in these quiet interludes that we can truly connect with ourselves and the world around us. Spiritual self-care is not about adhering to a particular belief system; rather, it's about nurturing your inner being, finding peace, and connecting with something greater than yourself. This chapter delves into practices that will help you cultivate a sense of spiritual well-being, even amidst the chaos of motherhood.

1. Embrace the Dawn: The early morning, when the world is still, offers a unique opportunity for reflection and meditation. Begin your day by waking up just a few minutes earlier than usual. Use this time to sit in silence, observe the sunrise, or simply breathe in the new day. This practice helps set a calm, centered tone for the day ahead.

2. Gratitude Journaling: Start or end your day by writing down three things you're grateful for. This simple act shifts your focus from what's lacking to what's abundant in your life. It can be as simple as a warm cup of coffee, a child's laughter, or the comfort of your bed. Over time, this practice cultivates an attitude of gratitude, enhancing your overall sense of well-being.

3. Walking Meditation: Combine exercise with spiritual practice through walking meditation. Choose a natural setting for your walk, like a park or a garden. As you walk, focus on the sensation of your feet touching the ground, the rhythm of your breath, and the sounds around you. This practice helps you stay present and grounded.

4. Create a Sacred Space: Dedicate a small area in your home as your sacred space. It can be a corner of a room with a comfortable chair, some candles, and perhaps a few inspirational books or objects. Spend a few minutes there each day meditating, praying, or simply sitting in quiet contemplation.

5. Nature Immersion: Regularly spend time in nature to reconnect with your spiritual self. Whether it's a hike in the woods, a walk on the beach, or simply sitting under a tree in your backyard, being in nature has a profound ability to soothe the soul and provide a sense of connectedness to the larger world.

6. Mindful Breathing: Practice mindful breathing to center yourself, especially during stressful moments. Take a few deep breaths, focusing solely on the act of breathing. Feel your chest rise and fall, and listen to the sound of your breath. This practice can be a quick and effective way to return to a state of calm and clarity.

7. Volunteer Work: Engaging in volunteer work can be a deeply fulfilling spiritual practice. It connects you with others, provides a sense of purpose, and offers perspective on your own life. Choose a cause that resonates with you and dedicate a few hours a month to this service.

8. Cultivate Compassion: Practice compassion towards yourself and others. This can be as simple as offering a kind word, a smile, or a helping hand. Being compassionate increases your empathy and connection to others, which is vital for spiritual growth.

9. Yoga for the Soul: Yoga is not just a physical exercise; it's a spiritual practice that harmonizes the body, mind, and spirit. Incorporate a gentle yoga routine into your week. Focus not just on the poses but also on the breath and the mindfulness aspect of the practice.

10. Spiritual Reading: Allocate some time each week for spiritual reading. This could be religious texts, philosophical works, or contemporary books on spirituality and personal growth. This practice can provide comfort, inspiration, and new perspectives on life.

11. Guided Meditation: Use guided meditations to explore different aspects of spirituality. There are numerous apps and online resources available, offering guided sessions on topics like peace, love, forgiveness, and gratitude. These can be particularly useful if you're new to meditation or if you find it challenging to quiet your mind.

12. Connect with a Community: Find a spiritual community that resonates with you, whether it's a church, temple, meditation group, or online forum. Being part of a community provides a sense of belonging and support as you explore your spiritual path.

13. Celebrate the Seasons: Acknowledge and celebrate the changing of the seasons. This can be through rituals, decorating your home, or simply observing the changes in nature. It's a way to stay connected to the earth's rhythm and recognize the impermanence of life.

14. Let Go of What Doesn't Serve You: Spiritual growth often involves letting go of things that hinder our progress. This could be negative thoughts, toxic relationships, or old grudges. Consciously releasing these frees up emotional space for more positive, nurturing experiences.

15. Practice Mindful Listening: Engage in mindful listening with your children, partner, or friends. This means fully focusing on the person speaking, without planning your response or judgment. Mindful listening enhances your relationships and fosters a deeper connection with others.

16. Express Your Creativity: Engage in creative activities like painting, writing, crafting, or gardening. Creative expression is a form of spiritual practice, allowing you to explore and express your inner self.

17. Reflective Evening Routine: End your day with a reflective routine. This could involve light stretching, reviewing the day's events, setting intentions for the next day, or a short meditation. This practice helps you wind down and prepare for restful sleep.

By integrating these spiritual self-care practices into your life, you can find pockets of peace and clarity amid the hustle and bustle of motherhood. Remember, the journey to inner peace is personal and ever-evolving. What resonates with you one day might change the next. The key is to stay open, curious, and forgiving as you explore these practices, allowing them to guide you to a deeper understanding and appreciation of your spiritual self.

Chapter 7: Physical Fitness and Energy

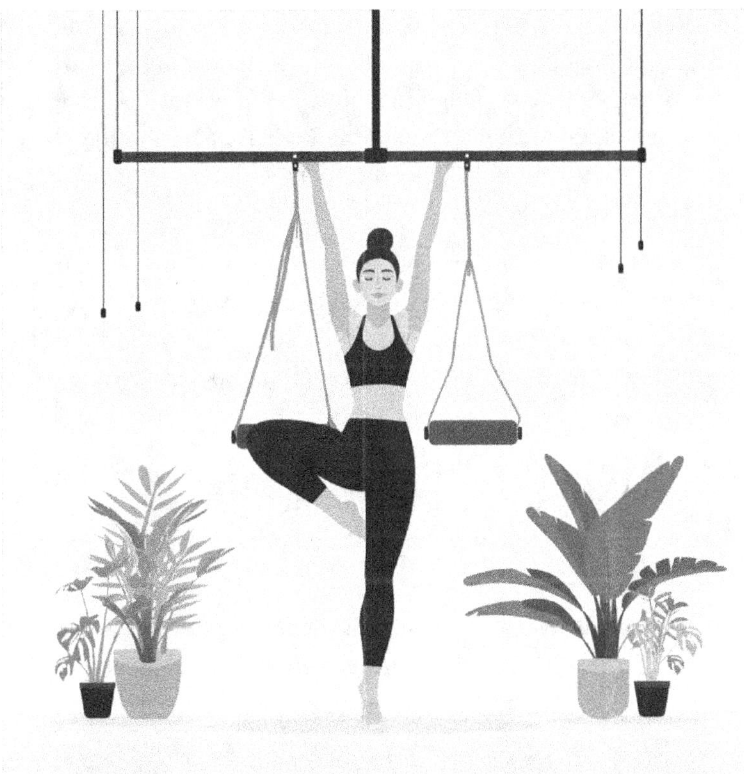

In the golden light of dawn, when the world seems to hold its breath in anticipation of the day ahead, lies the perfect moment for a busy mom to claim some time for herself. Physical fitness and energy are not just about maintaining a shape or achieving fitness goals; they're about nurturing your body's strength, vitality, and resilience, enabling you to meet the demands of motherhood with grace and vigor.

Integrating Movement into Daily Life

Embrace the Spontaneous Dance Party: Who says workouts need to be structured or done in a gym? Turn up your favorite tunes and have a dance party with your kids in the living room. Not only does it get your heart pumping, but it also brings joy and laughter into your home, creating lasting memories.

The Power of Ten: Find pockets of time for ten squats while waiting for the kettle to boil, ten lunges while brushing your teeth, or ten calf raises while reading a bedtime story. These micro-movements add up throughout the day, contributing significantly to your physical well-being without overwhelming your schedule.

Walk and Talk: Transform phone calls into walking meetings. Whether it's a catch-up with a friend or a work conference call, walking while talking keeps your body active and your mind engaged, turning a sedentary activity into a productive fitness session.

Stair Mastery: Choose the stairs over the elevator whenever possible. This simple switch is a powerful cardiovascular exercise that strengthens your legs and core, enhancing your stamina and endurance.

Active Commuting: If feasible, bike or walk your kids to school instead of driving. This not only incorporates physical activity into your daily routine but also sets a positive example for your children about the value of fitness and environmental consciousness.

Fun and Efficient Workouts for Moms

High-Intensity Interval Training (HIIT) at Home: HIIT workouts are perfect for busy moms because they pack maximum benefits into minimal time. A 20-minute session at home can be just as effective as an hour at the gym. Use bodyweight exercises like push-ups, burpees, and jumping jacks to get your heart rate up and build strength.

Yoga Flow for Flexibility and Strength: Yoga is not just a physical exercise; it's a practice that harmonizes body, mind, and spirit. A 15-minute yoga flow in the morning can increase your flexibility, strengthen your body, and prepare your mind for the day ahead with a sense of peace and focus.

Pilates for Core and Posture: Pilates exercises focus on core strength, flexibility, and overall body conditioning. Incorporating Pilates into your routine can improve your posture (a common concern for moms carrying little ones), enhance your flexibility, and build muscle tone.

Resistance Band Workouts: Resistance bands are affordable, portable, and versatile, making them an ideal fitness tool for home workouts. They can be used to add resistance to exercises, targeting specific muscle groups and increasing the effectiveness of your workouts without needing heavy equipment.

Family Bike Rides: Turn exercise into an adventure with family bike rides on the weekend. It's a wonderful way to explore your neighborhood or local parks while getting a great cardiovascular workout. Plus, it encourages outdoor activity and fitness as a family value.

Restorative Yoga Poses for Every Level

Child's Pose (Balasana): This pose is a haven of rest, offering a gentle stretch for the back, hips, and thighs while calming the mind and relieving stress. It's a grounding posture that busy moms can use to find a moment of tranquility amidst a chaotic day.

Cat-Cow Stretch (Marjaryasana-Bitilasana): This sequence gently massages the spine and belly organs while also serving as a calming breath exercise. It helps in releasing back tension and increasing spinal flexibility, making it ideal for moms who spend a lot of time lifting children or sitting.

Legs-Up-The-Wall Pose (Viparita Karani): This restorative pose is excellent for relieving tired legs and feet, improving circulation, and calming the nervous system. It's a simple yet powerful way to unwind at the end of the day, especially if you've been on your feet for long periods.

Supported Bridge Pose (Setu Bandhasana): Using a yoga block or a thick book under your lower back, this modified bridge pose helps alleviate stress in the back muscles, improve digestion, and reduce anxiety. It's a gentle way to open the chest and shoulders, areas often hunched over from carrying children or working at a computer.

Seated Forward Bend (Paschimottanasana): Ideal for stretching the spine, shoulders, and hamstrings, this pose also helps calm the brain and relieve stress. It can be particularly beneficial for moms looking for a quiet moment to reflect and stretch after a long day.

Physical fitness and energy are essential not just for the well-being of busy moms but for the entire family. By incorporating movement into daily life, engaging in fun and efficient workouts, and practicing restorative yoga poses, moms can build a foundation of physical strength and mental resilience. These activities not only enhance physical health but also provide valuable moments of joy, relaxation, and connection with oneself and loved ones.

Remember, the journey to maintaining your physical fitness and energy is not about perfection; it's about finding what works for you and your unique lifestyle. It's about making small, manageable changes that collectively make a significant impact on your well-being. As you navigate the beautiful chaos of motherhood, let these practices be a source of strength, joy, and vitality, empowering you to live each day with enthusiasm and grace.

Chapter 8: Creating Joyful Moments

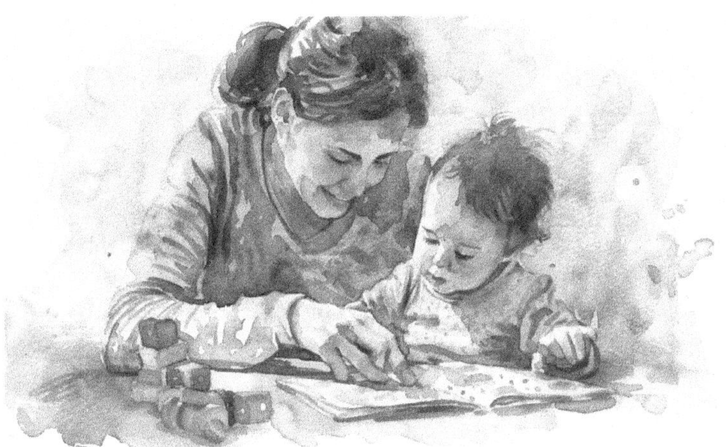

As the sun breaks through the early morning haze, a new day beckons, offering a canvas upon which to paint moments of joy, creativity, and connection. For busy moms, the quest for personal fulfillment and happiness often gets lost in the shuffle of daily responsibilities. Yet, it is within these precious moments of self-expression and adventure that we find our true essence and the vibrancy of life. This chapter is dedicated to the art of creating joyful moments through crafting, music, dance, and the simple pleasures of planning mini-adventures and staycations. Each activity is a thread in the tapestry of self-care, woven with the intention of bringing light, color, and energy back into your life.

Crafting and Creative Expression

1. Scrapbooking Life's Treasures: Begin with the simple joy of scrapbooking, a creative outlet that not only allows for artistic expression but also serves as a vessel for preserving memories. Set aside an hour each week to compile photographs, ticket stubs, and other memorabilia into a scrapbook. This practice isn't just about creating a beautiful album; it's a meditative process that allows you to reflect on joyful memories, fostering a sense of gratitude and contentment.

2. Painting as a Meditative Practice: Painting offers a way to express emotions and thoughts without words. Whether it's watercolor, acrylics, or digital painting, focus on the process rather than the outcome. Allow yourself to get lost in the colors and strokes, using this time as a meditative practice to quiet your mind and release stress.

3. DIY Home Decor Projects: Transform your living space with DIY home decor projects. From crafting homemade candles to creating wall art, these activities not only personalize your space but also provide a sense of accomplishment. Tackle one small project at a time, and involve your children if possible, turning it into a fun family activity.

4. Knitting and Crocheting for Mindfulness: The repetitive motion of knitting and crocheting has been shown to have a calming effect, similar to meditation. Start with simple patterns to create scarves, hats, or blankets. This practice can be especially rewarding as you see your work progress and come to fruition, offering both a creative outlet and practical results.

5. Writing and Illustrating a Personal Storybook: Channel your experiences, dreams, and lessons learned into writing and illustrating a personal storybook. This can be a fictional tale inspired by real-life events or a memoir of sorts. The act of writing is therapeutic, helping to process emotions and experiences, while illustrating adds a visual dimension to your narrative, making it uniquely yours.

Music and Dance: The Rhythm of Life

6. Creating a Personalized Playlist: Music has the power to uplift, heal, and inspire. Spend some time creating a personalized playlist filled with songs that spark joy, motivate you, or calm your mind. Let this playlist be your go-to during moments of self-care, whether you're relaxing, working out, or needing an emotional boost.

7. Exploring New Music Genres: Broaden your musical horizons by exploring new genres. Dedicate a week to immerse yourself in a genre you're unfamiliar with, whether it's classical, jazz, world music, or electronic. Discovering new sounds can be a refreshing way to find inspiration and awaken your senses.

8. Dance Like Nobody's Watching: Dancing is a wonderful way to express yourself and shake off stress. Have a solo dance party in your living room, letting loose to your favorite tunes. This activity is not about skill but about freedom of movement and the joy it brings. It's also a great way to get a fun workout.

9. Singing for the Soul: Singing, whether in the shower, car, or while doing chores, can be incredibly liberating. It's a way to express emotions and relieve stress. If you're feeling adventurous, join a local choir or take vocal lessons, embracing the communal joy and personal growth that comes with singing.

10. Learning to Play a Musical Instrument: Challenge yourself by learning to play a musical instrument. Whether it's the guitar, piano, ukulele, or even digital music production, the process of learning and creating music can be deeply rewarding. Dedicate a small amount of time each day to practice, and celebrate each milestone in your musical journey.

Planning Mini-Adventures and Staycations

11. Exploring Local Attractions: Often, we overlook the beauty and opportunities for adventure in our own backyards. Dedicate a day to explore local attractions you've never visited before. Whether it's a museum, park, hiking trail, or a historic site, approaching your local area with the curiosity of a tourist can reveal new and exciting experiences.

12. Themed Staycations at Home: Transform your home into a staycation paradise with a theme. This could be as simple as a spa day, where you pamper yourself with homemade beauty treatments, or as elaborate as turning your living room into a cinema for a movie marathon. Themes like "A Day in Paris" can inspire French cuisine cooking, watching French films, and even dressing the part.

13. Backyard Camping: For a change of scenery, try backyard camping. Set up a tent, prepare a campfire (safety permitting), and enjoy a night under the stars. It's a wonderful way to disconnect from technology and reconnect with nature, even if it's just a few steps from your home.

14. Virtual Travel Experiences: When physical travel isn't possible, virtual travel can offer a sense of escape and adventure. Many museums, zoos, and historical sites offer free virtual tours. Set aside an evening to "travel" to a new country via these tours, learning about different cultures and histories from the comfort of your home.

15. Crafting a Vision Board for Future Adventures: Finally, create a vision board for future adventures. Use magazines, printouts, and any other materials to visualize the places you'd like to visit and experiences you'd like to have. This not only serves as a creative outlet but also as a reminder of the exciting possibilities that await, motivating you to make those dreams a reality.

Creating joyful moments through crafting, music, dance, and mini-adventures is a testament to the endless possibilities for enrichment and fulfillment in our daily lives. Each of these activities offers a unique way to reconnect with ourselves, explore our creativity, and experience the world in new and meaningful ways. As busy moms, it's crucial to remember that self-care is not just about rest and relaxation but also about engaging in activities that bring us joy, stimulate our minds, and nourish our souls. By incorporating these practices into our self-care routine, we not only enhance our own well-being but also set a powerful example for our children on the importance of nurturing joy, creativity, and curiosity throughout life.

Chapter 9: Self-Care through Boundaries

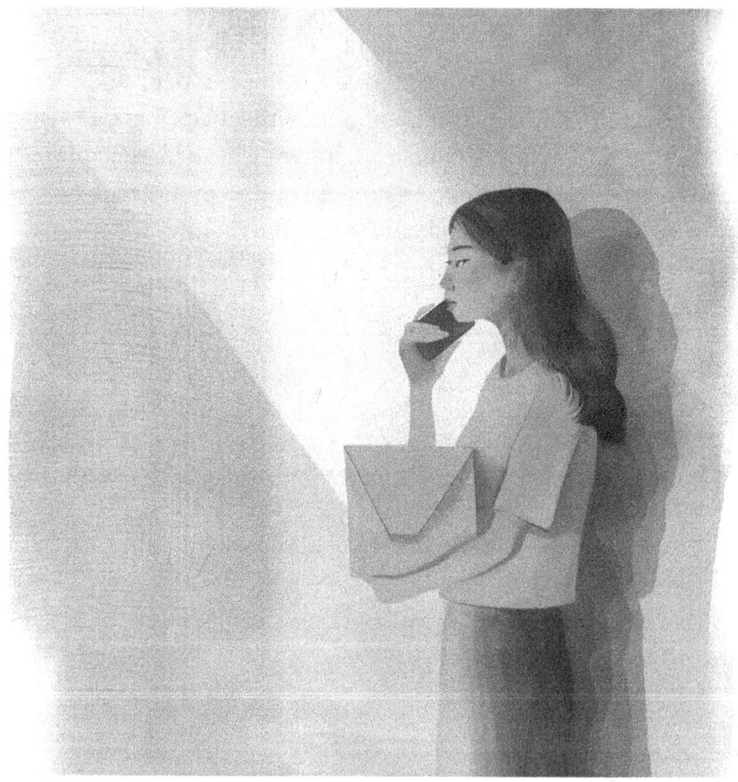

Amidst the whirlwind of motherhood, where time blurs into a mosaic of tasks, events, and emotions, setting boundaries emerges as an island of tranquility. It's a space where you can breathe, reflect, and realign with your core. This chapter is dedicated to teaching you the art of saying "no" with grace, balancing your needs against the demands of others, and managing your time effectively. Each of these aspects is a cornerstone of self-care, crucial for sustaining your energy, preserving your sanity, and nurturing your spirit.

The Graceful No

1. Understanding the Power of No: The first step in learning to say no is recognizing its value. No is not just a denial; it's an affirmation of your priorities, needs, and personal limits. It's a powerful tool for shaping your life according to your desires, rather than being swayed by the expectations of others.

2. Identifying When to Say No: Listen to your gut. If you feel dread, resentment, or overwhelm at the thought of adding another task to your plate, it's a sign that you should consider saying no. Your emotions are powerful indicators of your true capacity.

3. Communicating No with Empathy: Saying no doesn't mean you have to be harsh or uncaring. Frame your refusal around your current commitments or personal needs. For example, "I appreciate your thinking of me for this project, but I'm currently committed to priorities that require my full attention."

4. Offering Alternatives: When saying no, it can be helpful to offer an alternative. If you cannot commit to a request, suggest another person who might be interested or a future time when you might be available. This shows that while you're unable to fulfill the request now, you still value the relationship.

5. Practice Makes Perfect: Like any skill, saying no gracefully takes practice. Start small, with low-stakes situations, and gradually build up your confidence. Over time, you'll find it becomes easier, and the guilt associated with saying no will diminish.

Balancing Your Needs

6. Recognizing Your Worth: You are your most valuable asset. This realization is the bedrock of setting boundaries. Understanding and valuing your worth empowers you to make decisions that reflect your self-respect and commitment to self-care.

7. Prioritization is Key: Begin each day by identifying your top three priorities. These should align with your long-term goals and values. Everything else is secondary. This simple practice helps you to stay focused on what truly matters, making it easier to set boundaries around less critical tasks.

8. Learn to Delegate: Delegation is not a sign of weakness; it's a strategy for balance. By entrusting tasks to others, you free up your time and energy for activities that are more meaningful or require your unique skills. Remember, it's about working smarter, not harder.

9. Setting Limits with Technology: In an always-connected world, it's vital to set boundaries around your use of technology. Designate tech-free times, particularly during family meals, before bedtime, and during personal relaxation moments. This not only reduces stress but also models healthy behavior for your children.

10. Self-Care Appointments: Treat self-care activities as non-negotiable appointments. Whether it's a 15-minute meditation session, a weekly yoga class, or a monthly massage, schedule these activities with the same seriousness as you would a doctor's appointment. This mindset shift ensures that self-care remains a priority.

Time Management Strategies

11. The Magic of the Morning Routine: Start your day with intention by establishing a morning routine dedicated to self-care. Even 15 minutes spent in meditation, journaling, or exercise can set a positive tone for the day ahead.

12. The Pomodoro Technique: This time management method involves working for 25 minutes, then taking a 5-minute break. It's particularly effective for tasks you're dreading. The short bursts of work feel more manageable, and the frequent breaks keep your mind fresh.

13. Time Blocking: Allocate specific blocks of time for different activities or tasks throughout your day. This includes work, family time, and self-care. Time blocking helps prevent tasks from bleeding into each other, reducing stress and increasing productivity.

14. The Two-Minute Rule: If a task takes less than two minutes, do it immediately. This rule helps keep small tasks from piling up, which can become overwhelming over time. It's a simple strategy that can significantly improve your daily efficiency.

15. Weekly Planning Sessions: Dedicate time each week to plan the week ahead. Outline key tasks, appointments, and self-care activities. This not only provides a clear roadmap for the week but also helps you identify potential challenges and adjust your plan accordingly.

16. Learning to Adjust: Flexibility is a critical component of time management. Despite our best plans, life happens. When unexpected events arise, give yourself permission to adjust your plans. This adaptability reduces stress and allows you to maintain a balance between your needs and the demands of the moment.

17. Celebrating Small Wins: Take time to acknowledge and celebrate your achievements, no matter how small. This practice fosters a sense of accomplishment and motivates you to continue setting and respecting your boundaries.

By embracing these strategies, you can transform your approach to self-care through the establishment of healthy boundaries. It's about recognizing your limits, valuing your own needs, and managing your time in a way that honors your well-being. Remember, setting boundaries is not selfish; it's a fundamental aspect of self-care that enables you to be the best version of yourself, for you and for those you love.

Chapter 10: Personal Growth and Self-Discovery

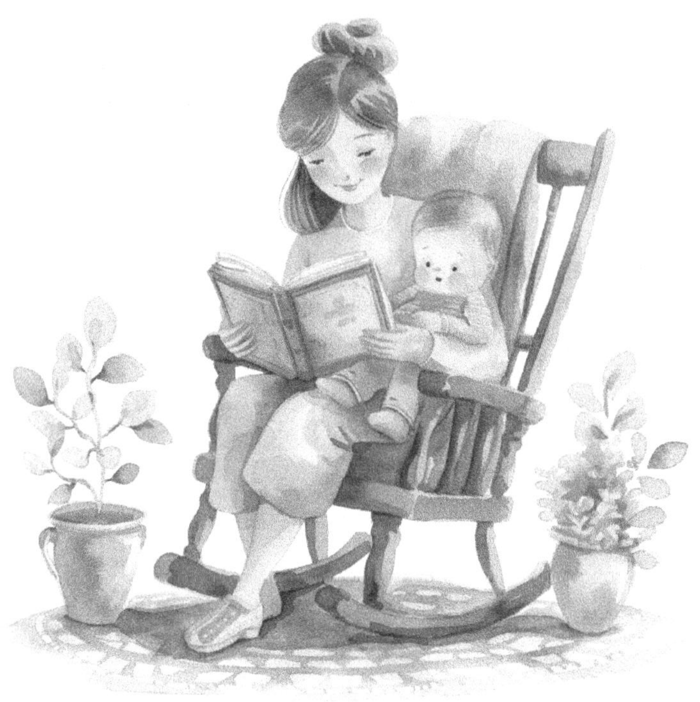

In the quiet moments of the early morning, when the world is still asleep, and you find yourself alone with your thoughts, it's an opportune time to reflect on who you are and who you wish to become. Personal growth and self-discovery are journeys that many of us embark on but often, as busy moms, we sideline these quests in favor of immediate family needs. However, nurturing your own growth is not just a gift to yourself but to those you love, for as you evolve, so too does the quality of your presence and care for others.

Setting and Pursuing Personal Goals

1. **Identify What Truly Matters:** Start by reflecting on what aspects of your life you wish to improve or change. Is it your health, your career, your personal skills, or perhaps your relationships? Write down areas that resonate most deeply with you, no matter how big or small they may seem.

2. **SMART Goals:** Once you have identified your areas for growth, set SMART (Specific, Measurable, Achievable, Relevant, Time-bound) goals. For instance, instead of a vague goal like "I want to be healthier," a SMART goal would be, "I will walk 30 minutes a day, five days a week, for the next three months."

3. **Break It Down:** Large goals can be overwhelming. Break them down into smaller, actionable steps. If your goal is to change careers, start with updating your resume, then move on to networking, and so on.

4. **Celebrate Small Wins:** Every step forward is a victory. Celebrate these moments to motivate yourself further. Small rewards for small achievements can keep the momentum going.

5. **Seek Support:** Share your goals with friends, family, or a mentor who can offer support, advice, and accountability.

Embracing Change and New Beginnings

6. **Cultivate a Growth Mindset:** View challenges as opportunities to learn rather than insurmountable obstacles. A growth mindset encourages resilience and adaptability, essential qualities for navigating life's inevitable changes.

7. **Letting Go of Fear:** Fear of failure can be a significant barrier to personal growth. Acknowledge your fears, but don't let them dictate your actions. Remember, every attempt, successful or not, is a step toward growth.

8. **Embrace Uncertainty:** Change often comes with uncertainty, which can be uncomfortable. Embrace it as a part of the growth process. Uncertainty means you're moving beyond your comfort zone, a space where personal transformation occurs.

9. **New Beginnings as Opportunities:** Whether it's a new job, moving to a new city, or starting a new hobby, view each beginning as an opportunity to learn and grow. Each new start is a chance to redefine and rediscover yourself.

10. **Stay Open to Learning:** Personal growth is a lifelong journey. Stay open to learning from every experience and person you encounter. Every lesson is an opportunity to grow.

Self-Compassion: Treating Yourself with Kindness

11. **Practice Self-Compassion:** Be as kind to yourself as you would be to a dear friend. Recognize that being imperfect is part of being human. When you stumble, offer yourself understanding and kindness instead of harsh self-criticism.

12. **Mindful Acceptance:** Practice mindfulness to stay present with your experiences without judgment. Acknowledging your feelings and thoughts without criticism can lead to greater emotional equilibrium and self-acceptance.

13. **Speak Kindly to Yourself:** Pay attention to your inner dialogue. Replace negative self-talk with positive affirmations. Instead of saying, "I can't do this," try, "I'm doing my best, and that's all I can ask of myself."

14. **Nurture Your Needs:** Recognize and honor your needs, whether they're for rest, play, social interaction, or solitude. Neglecting your needs can lead to burnout and resentment, which hinder personal growth.

15. **Forgive Yourself:** Forgiveness is a powerful aspect of self-compassion. Forgive yourself for past mistakes.

Understanding that errors are part of the learning process allows you to move forward with grace.

Implementing Your Personal Growth Plan

16. **Create a Vision Board:** A visual representation of your goals can serve as a daily reminder and inspiration. Include images, quotes, and anything else that resonates with your aspirations.

17. **Journal Your Journey:** Keep a journal of your thoughts, feelings, successes, and setbacks. Writing provides clarity and perspective, helping you navigate your path to personal growth.

18. **Regular Check-ins:** Set aside time weekly or monthly to review your progress. What's working? What's not? Adjust your strategies as needed.

19. **Stay Flexible:** Be prepared to adjust your goals as you grow and as circumstances change. Flexibility is key to sustainable growth.

20. **Practice Gratitude:** Regularly reflect on what you're grateful for. Gratitude shifts your focus from what you lack to the abundance you already have, fostering a positive mindset that nurtures growth.

In the pursuit of personal growth and self-discovery, it's essential to remember that the journey itself is more important than the destination. Each step, each realization, and each moment of self-compassion is a testament to your commitment to becoming the best version of yourself—not just for your own well-being but for the enrichment of your family's life as well. Embracing change, setting meaningful goals, and treating yourself with kindness and compassion are not just pathways to personal growth; they're acts of love that ripple outwards, impacting everyone around you.

As you embark on this journey, remember that personal growth is not a linear process. There will be days of profound insight and days where progress seems all but invisible. Yet, it's these very fluctuations that make the journey so enriching. Each day offers a new opportunity to learn, to grow, and to explore the vast landscape of your inner world. By committing to this path, you're not only fostering your own development but also modeling a life of continuous learning and self-compassion for your children.

In the quietude of the night, when you finally have a moment to pause and reflect, consider the vastness of your journey. You've ventured through the trials and triumphs of motherhood, each step an act of immense love and dedication. Now, as you turn the pages of your own story, exploring the chapters of personal growth and self-discovery, remember that this, too, is a profound act of love—a love for yourself that is as vital and nourishing as the care you extend to others.

Your journey of personal growth and self-discovery is a beautiful, winding path filled with lessons of strength, resilience, and boundless love. It's a testament to the incredible capacity for transformation that resides within you. As you continue to explore, learn, and grow, know that each step forward enriches not only your life but also the lives of those you hold dear. This journey, with all its challenges and joys, is a celebration of you—your strengths, your dreams, your potential. And as you move forward, embracing each new day with courage and kindness, remember that the most profound growth often comes from the simplest acts of self-care and self-compassion.

Chapter 11: Nurturing Relationships

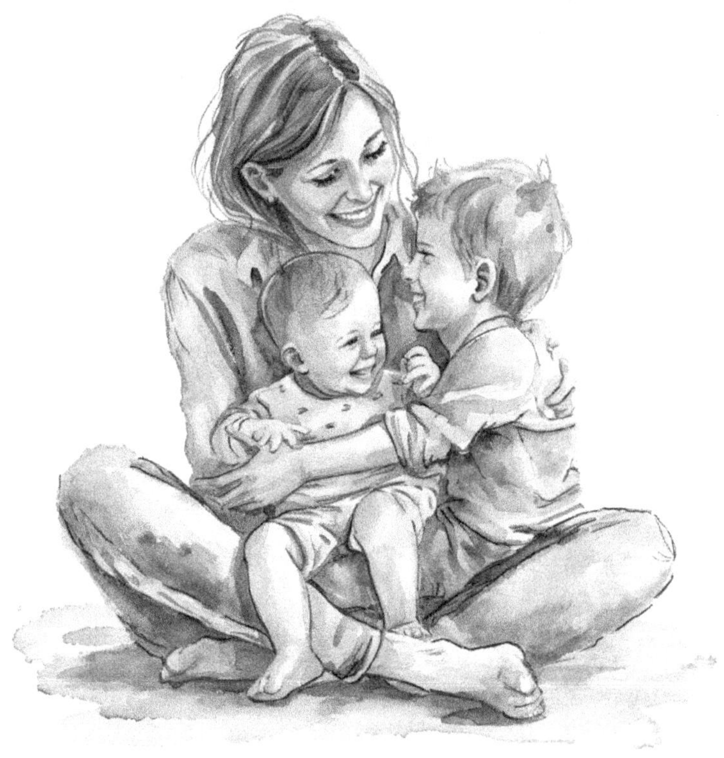

In the heart of a bustling kitchen, amidst the symphony of early morning routines, lies the unspoken language of love and connection that binds families together. As busy moms, we often find ourselves caught in the whirlwind of daily tasks, forgetting that the essence of our lives is not in the to-dos but in the to-loves. Nurturing relationships with our partners, children, and friends isn't just another item on our checklist; it's the cornerstone of a fulfilling life and an integral part of self-care.

Partner Connection Activities (5 Practices)

1. Weekly Date Nights - At Home or Out: Commit to a weekly date night with your partner, alternating who plans the evening. It doesn't have to be elaborate; simplicity often breeds intimacy. One week, it might be a movie night at home with homemade popcorn. The next, a quiet dinner at a local restaurant. The key is undivided attention, away from the hustle of parenting duties, to reconnect and strengthen your bond.

2. Communication Rituals: Establish a daily check-in ritual, perhaps over a cup of coffee in the morning or a quiet moment after the kids are in bed. Use this time to share your thoughts, feelings, and dreams. Active listening plays a crucial role here—this isn't about problem-solving but about understanding and empathizing with each other.

3. Shared Hobbies: Find a hobby or activity you both enjoy and dedicate time to pursue it together. Whether it's gardening, biking, cooking, or painting, shared hobbies offer a unique way to connect and create joyful memories, reinforcing your partnership outside of your roles as parents.

4. Love Letters or Notes: Rediscover the lost art of writing love letters or notes. A simple "I appreciate you" note tucked into a work bag or a heartfelt letter on an anniversary can make a significant impact. It's a tangible reminder of your affection and appreciation for one another.

5. Relationship Goals Setting: Once a year, sit down together to set relationship goals. These could range from financial planning, personal growth, to bucket list adventures. Setting goals together not only strengthens your bond but also ensures you're both moving in the same direction, with shared aspirations and dreams.

Family Bonding Activities (5 Practices)

1. Family Meetings: Hold weekly family meetings to discuss upcoming events, any issues or concerns, and to plan fun activities. This fosters open communication, teaches problem-solving skills, and makes every family member feel valued and heard.

2. Cook and Eat Together: Make meal preparation a family affair. Assign tasks to each family member, from picking recipes to setting the table. This not only teaches valuable life skills but also creates a sense of teamwork and belonging.

3. One-on-One Time: Schedule individual dates with each child, allowing them to choose the activity. This special time is crucial in understanding their unique personalities and interests, strengthening your bond, and showing them they are valued as individuals.

4. Volunteer as a Family: Choose a cause or a community service project to support as a family. Volunteering teaches compassion, empathy, and the importance of giving back, all while spending quality time together.

5. Bedtime Rituals: End each day with a consistent bedtime ritual. Whether it's reading a story, sharing the highs and lows of the day, or simply cuddling, this precious time creates a comforting routine and deepens your connection.

Friendship Nurturing Tips (5 Practices)

1. Scheduled Friend Dates: Just as you would with your partner, schedule regular meet-ups with friends. It could be a monthly brunch, a book club, or a walking group. Consistency helps maintain these important connections.

2. Support Each Other's Interests: Show interest in and support for your friends' hobbies and achievements. Attend their events, celebrate their successes, and encourage their endeavors. This mutual support is the backbone of a strong friendship.

3. Group Chats or Social Media Groups: Stay connected through technology. A group chat or a private social media group can keep the conversation going, even when you can't meet in person. Share updates, jokes, or words of encouragement.

4. Offer Help, Ask for Help: Be proactive in offering help during their times of need, and don't hesitate to ask for help when you're the one in need. This exchange strengthens bonds and builds a supportive network.

5. Remember Special Occasions: Make an effort to remember and celebrate friends' special occasions, whether with a card, a call, or a thoughtful gift. It's a simple gesture that can mean the world to someone.

Nurturing Relationships: The Keystone of Self-Care

In the tapestry of life, relationships form the threads that hold us together, providing strength, comfort, and vibrant colors. As busy moms, we might think of self-care in terms of solitude and personal activities, but at its core, self-care is also about the quality of our connections with those around us. It's about finding balance, sharing love, and building a community that uplifts and supports us.

Nurturing our relationships requires intention and effort, but the rewards are immeasurable. Strong connections not only enhance our well-being but also model the importance of relationships to our children. They learn how to communicate, show empathy, and build their own relationships based on the examples we set.

As we journey through the myriad responsibilities of motherhood, let's remember that taking care of our relationships is as vital as taking care of our health. It's in the laughter shared with a partner, the quiet conversations with a child, and the comforting presence of a friend that we find our deepest joy and fulfillment.

In embracing these practices, we not only enrich our lives but also create a legacy of love and connection for generations to come. The art of nurturing relationships is, ultimately, the art of nurturing ourselves.

Chapter 12: Building a Self-Care Routine

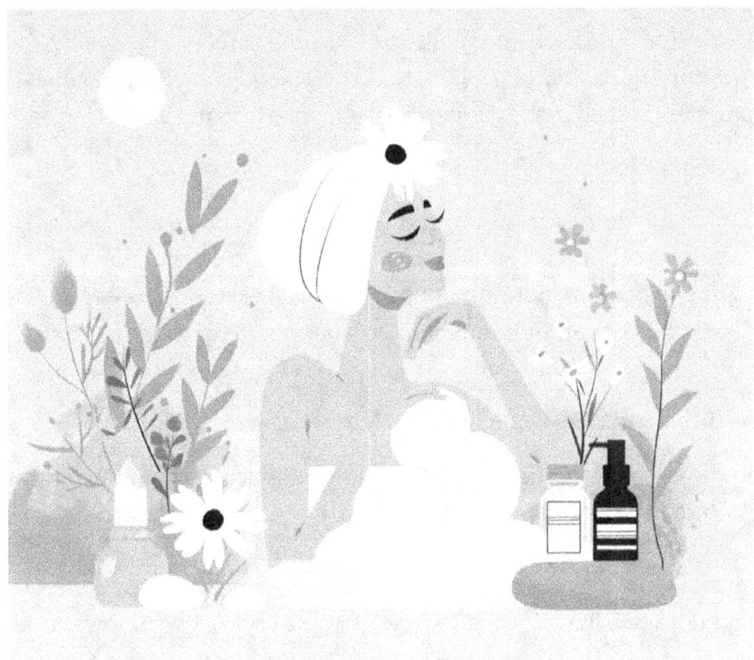

Building a self-care routine is akin to weaving a tapestry of practices that color our days with peace, strength, and joy. This chapter is dedicated to guiding you in designing your ideal self-care routine, navigating the inevitable obstacles, and celebrating each step forward, no matter how small.

Designing Your Ideal Self-Care Routine

Creating a Blueprint for Well-being

Begin by envisioning your ideal day. What activities fill you with energy? Which moments of stillness bring you peace? Your self-care routine should be a reflection of what truly resonates with your soul. Consider the various dimensions of self-care we've explored: physical, emotional, mental, and spiritual. Aim to incorporate elements from each dimension to create a balanced routine.

1. Start Small and Specific

Choose one or two practices to start. It could be as simple as a five-minute morning meditation or writing three things you're grateful for each night. The key is consistency; even the smallest practices, when done regularly, can have profound effects.

2. Schedule Your Self-Care

Treat your self-care time with the same importance as a doctor's appointment or a parent-teacher conference. By scheduling it, you're making a commitment to yourself. Use tools at your disposal, like setting reminders on your phone or marking it on your family calendar.

3. Integrate Self-Care Into Daily Activities

Look for opportunities to incorporate self-care into your existing routine. Turn your shower into a spa-like experience with aromatherapy, or practice mindfulness while drinking your morning coffee. These moments of care can become seamless parts of your day.

4. Build a Self-Care Kit

Assemble a small collection of items that aid your self-care practices. This could be a journal, a favorite tea, essential oils, or a yoga mat. Having these items readily available makes it easier to engage in your routine.

Overcoming Obstacles to Self-Care

Recognizing and Addressing Common Barriers

The path to consistent self-care is often littered with obstacles, from time constraints to feelings of guilt. Recognizing these barriers is the first step to overcoming them.

1. Time Constraints

For busy moms, finding time is a perpetual challenge. Look for hidden opportunities in your day, such as the early morning before others wake up or during lunch breaks. Remember, self-care doesn't have to be time-consuming. Even short periods are beneficial.

2. Feeling Guilty

Many moms struggle with guilt over taking time for themselves. It's crucial to reframe self-care as not only beneficial to you but also to your family. When you're well-cared-for, you're more present, patient, and joyful with your loved ones.

3. Lack of Support

If you're facing resistance or lack of support from family, communicate the importance of your self-care routine. Share how it improves your well-being and, by extension, benefits your family. Don't hesitate to ask for help or delegate tasks to make space for your self-care.

4. Staying Motivated

Motivation can wane, especially when results aren't immediately visible. Keep a journal to reflect on how your self-care practices impact your mood and energy levels. This can serve as a powerful reminder of their value.

Celebrating Progress and Embracing Imperfections

Acknowledging Every Step

Each action you take towards incorporating self-care into your life is an achievement. Celebrate the small victories, whether it's sticking to your routine for a week or simply taking a few deep breaths on a hectic day.

1. Create a Reward System

Build incentives for maintaining your routine. After a month of consistent self-care, treat yourself to something special, like a new book or a day out. These rewards not only offer motivation but also reinforce the idea that caring for yourself is a priority.

2. Share Your Journey

Connecting with other moms on a similar path can be incredibly rewarding. Share your successes and challenges, and celebrate each other's progress. This sense of community can provide encouragement and accountability.

3. Adjust as Needed

Your needs and circumstances will evolve, and so should your self-care routine. Regularly assess what's working and what isn't. Don't be afraid to adjust your practices to better suit your current life phase.

4. Embrace Imperfection

There will be days when your self-care routine falls by the wayside, and that's okay. The goal is progress, not perfection. Embrace these moments with kindness and remind yourself that every day is a new opportunity to prioritize your well-being.

As you embark on this journey of building and maintaining your self-care routine, remember that it's not about adding another item to your to-do list. It's about creating a life that feels good from the inside out. It's about showing up for yourself with the same love and dedication you give so freely to others. And most importantly, it's about recognizing that you, dear mom, are worthy of your own care.

Through the tapestry of practices you weave into your days, may you find the strength to meet challenges with grace, the courage to pursue your passions, and the peace to savor the precious moments of motherhood. Your self-care journey is a testament to the belief that by nurturing ourselves, we nurture our families and communities, creating ripples of well-being that touch the lives of those we love.

In embracing your essence and prioritizing your well-being, you not only reclaim your vitality but also model the importance of self-care to your children. You teach them that caring for oneself is not an act of selfishness but a fundamental aspect of living a balanced and fulfilling life.

Let this chapter serve as a compass to guide you in crafting a self-care routine that resonates with your unique spirit. As you navigate the complexities of motherhood, may your self-care practices be a beacon of light, illuminating the path to a more joyful, peaceful, and vibrant existence. Remember, the journey of self-care is continuous, with each day offering a new canvas upon which to paint your moments of care.

Final Word: A Journey Embraced

In the quiet moments of reflection, as the chapters of this book draw to a close, let us pause and look back on the journey we've embarked upon together. **"Embrace Your Essence: 101 Self-Care Practices for Busy Moms"** began as a guide, but has blossomed into something far more profound - a journey of rediscovery, resilience, and renewal.

As you stand at this juncture, with the insights and practices gleaned from these pages, you are not merely a reader; you are an explorer who has traversed the varied landscapes of self-care. You've delved into the depths of your own needs, experimented with nourishing practices, and faced the challenges of integrating self-care into the bustling life of motherhood.

This journey, however, does not end here. Rather, it transforms, evolves, and continues to unfold with each passing day. Self-care is not a destination but a path that winds and turns, offering new vistas and challenges. It is a lifelong commitment to yourself, a promise to honor and nurture your well-being amidst the myriad roles you play.

Embracing the Essence of You

At the heart of this journey is you – a remarkable, multifaceted individual with dreams, desires, and strengths. Remember, self-care is not selfish; it is essential. By taking care of yourself, you are better equipped to care for those you love. You become a beacon of strength, love, and balance, inspiring those around you.

The Ripple Effect of Self-Care

Your journey into self-care extends beyond the personal. It has the power to touch the lives of those around you – your family, friends, and community. By modeling self-care, you encourage others to embark on their own journeys of well-being. This creates a ripple effect, fostering a culture where self-care is understood, valued, and practiced.

The Ever-Changing Tapestry of Life

Life is an ever-changing tapestry, woven with threads of joy, challenge, love, and growth. Your self-care practices will need to adapt to the changing patterns of this tapestry. There will be times when your routine flows seamlessly, and times when it feels like an uphill battle. In both, there is learning and growth. Embrace these changes with grace and patience.

Celebrating Each Step

Every effort you make in nurturing yourself, no matter how small, is a victory. Celebrate these moments. Whether it's taking five minutes to breathe deeply, enjoying a quiet walk, or simply saying no to an overwhelming commitment, these acts of self-care are triumphs worth acknowledging.

A Continuous Path of Learning

As you move forward, remain open to learning and exploring new facets of self-care. This book is a foundation, but your journey is enriched by your experiences, experiments, and discoveries. Keep seeking, trying, and growing.

Your Story, Your Strength

Finally, remember that your story, with its unique challenges and triumphs, is your strength. Share it when you can, listen to others, and build a community that uplifts and supports. Together, we can shift the narrative around motherhood to one that includes and prioritizes the well-being of moms.

As you close this book, know that you are not closing the chapter on self-care. Instead, you are stepping forward with a toolkit of practices, a heart full of courage, and a spirit ready to embrace whatever lies ahead. Carry these lessons and insights with you, let them light your path, and continue to Embrace Your Essence, dear reader, for in doing so, you embrace the very joy of life itself.

Thank you for allowing this book to be a part of your journey. May it always be a source of inspiration and comfort as you navigate the beautiful, complex journey of motherhood and self-care.

Appendix: Takeaways List

As you turn the pages of this book and integrate its wisdom into your life, this appendix serves as a quick reference guide - a collection of key takeaways and distilled wisdom from each chapter. Use it as a beacon to guide you back to the core lessons and practices that resonate most with you.

Introduction: Awakening to Self-Care

- Self-care is essential, not optional, for busy moms.

- Overcoming guilt and societal pressures is key to embracing self-care.

- Self-care is a journey of rediscovery and empowerment.

Chapter 1: The Foundation of Self-Care

- Self-care encompasses physical, emotional, mental, and spiritual needs.

- Creating a personal self-care plan is the first step in this journey.

- Self-awareness is crucial in identifying your unique self-care needs.

Chapter 2: Quick Wins for Busy Days

- Incorporate simple mindfulness techniques to find calm amidst chaos.

- Deep breathing exercises can be a quick stress reliever.

- Short stretch routines can boost energy and improve physical well-being.

Chapter 3: Nourishing Your Body

- Healthy eating can be simplified and integrated into a busy schedule.

- Adequate hydration is key to maintaining energy and health.

- Establishing sleep rituals can significantly improve restorative sleep.

Chapter 4: Cultivating Emotional Resilience

- Journaling can aid in emotional clarity and strength.

- Building a supportive community is essential for emotional resilience.

- Developing stress and anxiety management techniques is crucial.

Chapter 5: Fostering Mental Well-Being

- Daily mindfulness practices enhance mental clarity and peace.

- Regular digital detoxes can improve mental health.

- Engaging in lifelong learning keeps the mind active and healthy.

Chapter 6: Spiritual Self-Care for Inner Peace

- Finding moments of solitude can recharge and refresh the spirit.

- Practicing gratitude can transform perspective and increase happiness.

- Connecting with nature can be a powerful spiritual practice.

Chapter 7: Physical Fitness and Energy

- Integrating movement into daily life boosts physical and mental health.

- Efficient workouts can fit into a busy mom's schedule.

- Yoga can be a restorative practice for all fitness levels.

Chapter 8: Creating Joyful Moments

- Creative expression is a joyful and therapeutic self-care practice.

- Music and dance can lift spirits and provide a fun escape.

- Planning mini-adventures and staycations can create lasting family memories.

Chapter 9: Self-Care through Boundaries

- Saying no is a powerful form of self-care.

- Balancing personal needs with family responsibilities is crucial.

- Effective delegation and time management can free up self-care time.

Chapter 10: Personal Growth and Self-Discovery

- Setting personal goals is a form of self-care that fosters growth.

- Embracing change can lead to new beginnings and self-discovery.

- Practicing self-compassion is essential for personal well-being.

Chapter 11: Nurturing Relationships

- Strengthening bonds with partners and children enhances family life.

- Cultivating friendships is important for emotional support.

- The act of giving and receiving love is a powerful self-care practice.

Chapter 12: Building a Self-Care Routine

- Designing a self-care routine requires planning and commitment.

- Overcoming obstacles to self-care is part of the journey.

- Celebrating progress, no matter how small, is important.

Epilogue: A Continuous Journey

- Self-care is an ongoing, evolving process.

- Staying committed to self-care practices is a lifelong endeavor.

- Inspiring others through your self-care journey is a powerful gift.

This appendix is not just a summary; it's a reminder that the practices and insights you've gained from this book are always within reach. As you navigate the complexities and joys of motherhood, let these takeaways be your guideposts, helping you stay aligned with your self-care journey and reminding you of the profound impact it has on your life and the lives of those you love. Remember, each step you take in caring for yourself is a step towards a more fulfilled, balanced, and joyful life.

Appendix: Quick Self-Care Checklist

In the rush of daily life, it can be challenging to remember all the different ways you can practice self-care. This quick checklist is designed to be a handy reference for busy moms. Whether you have a few minutes or an hour, these simple practices can help you recharge and find balance. You can return to this list whenever you need a reminder or inspiration.

Moments for Yourself

- ☐ Take three deep, calming breaths
- ☐ Stretch your body for five minutes
- ☐ Sip a cup of your favorite tea or coffee mindfully
- ☐ Write down three things you're grateful for
- ☐ Read a page or two of an inspiring book
- ☐ Apply your favorite lotion or perfume
- ☐ Spend a few minutes in the sun

Nourishing Your Body

- ☐ Drink a glass of water
- ☐ Eat a healthy snack (fruits, nuts, yogurt)
- ☐ Take a brisk 10-minute walk
- ☐ Do a quick yoga or Pilates routine
- ☐ Prepare a nutritious meal for yourself
- ☐ Have a mini dance session to your favorite song

Emotional and Mental Well-being

- ☐ Journal for five minutes

- [ ] Call or text a friend
- [ ] Watch a funny video to laugh
- [ ] Practice a five-minute mindfulness meditation
- [ ] Write down a positive affirmation and repeat it
- [ ] Spend time with a pet

Spiritual Self-Care

- [ ] Spend a few minutes in nature
- [ ] Meditate or pray
- [ ] Light a candle and reflect quietly
- [ ] Read or listen to a motivational podcast
- [ ] Practice deep breathing exercises
- [ ] Engage in a creative activity (drawing, crafting)

Relationships and Social Life

- [ ] Hug a loved one
- [ ] Play a game with your child
- [ ] Have a meaningful conversation with a partner or friend
- [ ] Plan a future outing with friends
- [ ] Join a community or a club that interests you

Personal Growth

- [ ] Set a goal for the week
- [ ] Learn something new (a recipe, a skill)
- [ ] Reflect on your recent achievements
- [ ] Plan a personal project
- [ ] Take a step towards a long-term goal

Physical Environment

☐ Organize a small area of your home

☐ Light a scented candle or use an essential oil diffuser

☐ Put on some comforting background music

☐ Declutter your workspace

☐ Create a cozy nook for relaxation

Routine and Rituals

☐ Establish a morning or evening routine

☐ Schedule your self-care time

☐ Create a weekly self-care plan

☐ Track your self-care activities

☐ Adjust your routine as needed

This checklist is not exhaustive but offers a variety of options to cater to different needs and time constraints. Feel free to adapt these suggestions to fit your lifestyle and preferences. Remember, the goal of self-care is to find practices that rejuvenate and empower you. Use this checklist as a starting point to explore what works best for you and embrace the journey of self-care with an open heart and mind.

www.ingramcontent.com/pod-product-compliance
Lightning Source LLC
Chambersburg PA
CBHW070958250726
48663CB00002B/285